How to Pop a Zit:
An Aesthetician's Guide to Safe "Popping"

Mahatmama.com is an imprint of RMedia.

ISBN: 1440425019

Table of Contents

The Expert

An Aesthetician is a person trained to administer topical skin-care treatments, advise customers on make-up and the care of skin and facial hair. An Aesthetician is trained in school to understand the workings of the skin and to be able to provide non-damaging assistance to individuals in the care of their skin.

Additionally an Aesthetician is trained to perform treatments on the epidermal layer of the skin. A Dermatologist is a medical professional who treats all layers of the skin, from the epidermis to the dermal layer.

Rupa Vickers Russell is a North Carolina State Board Certified Aesthetician. Her focus on skin care is to maintain a natural balance in the care of skin. Drawing from ancient skin care knowledge and integrating useful modern technologies, Ms. Russell practices as an Aesthetician in Florida and NC.

The Problem

What IS a Zit?

Pimple. Zit. Blackhead. Pustule. All these words describe one of the most unpleasant skin conditions people can suffer. It's annoying, it's unsightly and sometimes painful. Technically a Zit or pimple is the same as a pustule or blackhead. However a pustule is not a blackhead, or what professionals refer to as a comedone.

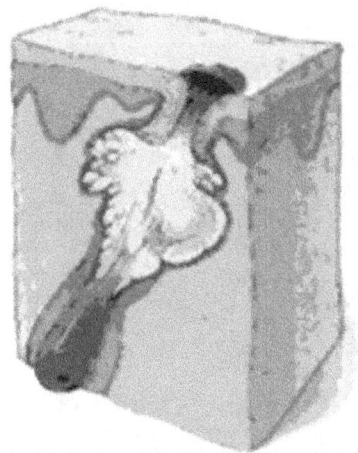

Comedone/Blackhead

A comedone is a pore that is clogged by debris. Generally it is a build up of sweat, dead skin and pollution or grit and grime that gets trapped in the orifice of the pore. But the key to a comedone or blackhead is that the pore can still breathe. The stuff is still trapped inside, but it's not covered by a layer of skin, or a cap. If the pore is filled with debris AND is covered by a layer of skin, then you've got yourself a pustule.

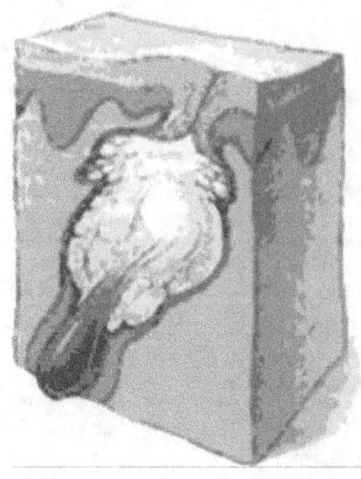

Whitehead

A whitehead is a pore that is impacted with debris, has a covering of skin, or a cap, but has not yet had an overabundance of white blood cells swell to the area. Often times this form of a zit is red and swollen, but doesn't have as large a white head as a pustule.

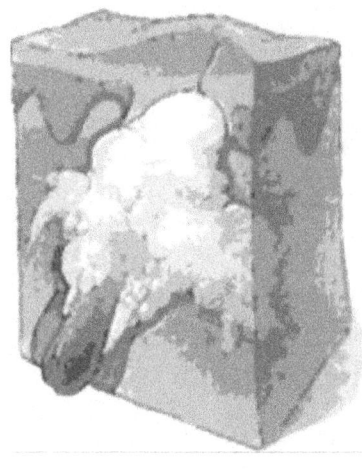

Pustule

A pustule is a pore that has something clogged inside of it, but there is skin covering the pore, a cap, which keeps the pore from breathing and therefore the trapped grime and Bacteria inside the pore overproduce and cause the skin tissue to become inflamed with a swell of white blood cells that the body sends to fight the dirt. This response, called pus, creates an unsightly pustule with an enlarged white head.

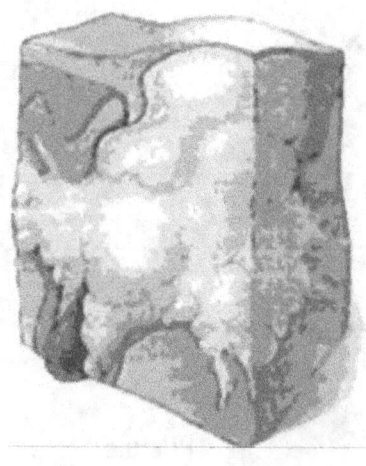

Cyst

If the bacterial infection runs deep inside the shaft of the pore, you could have a cyst on your hands. The problem with a cyst is that manual extraction (or picking or pressing) will not work The infection is deep enough and curvy enough that the only option is to allow your natural immune response to kick in and fight the debris, or to see a doctor and probably go on an antibiotic. If damaged, by improper picking or care, a cyst may only be removed with surgical intervention.

Good News

The good news is that your skin, and body, doesn't like having debris in it, so if your immune response is strong enough, and can beat the bacteria, then the skin will slowly but surely (usually 8-10 days for the ugly stage) win the battle and give you an easily extractable plug to remove from the pore. But that takes patience and confidence, because it'll be ugly until you can get it out. To boost your immune system, contact a nutritionist to get recommendations about immune building vitamins.

How did I get it?

There are many ways to cause a clogged pore. Usually maintaining a proper cleansing routine will help keep debris from off the skin. But all skin can from time to time suffer from a compacted pore. Once a pore becomes compacted with debris it can become a blackhead or become the more inflamed pustule.

Additionally diet does matter, but not the way you may think. You're not going to get a zit because you had a chocolate candy bar. But, if you eat the candy bar, and the rest of your diet is out of whack for your body, then the hormones in your system will adjust and this, this alone MAY stimulate an overproduction of oil, which if the conditions are right with cleanliness and bacteria presence, may contribute to the production of a zit.

Zit or Acne?

An occasional zit or blackhead is very different from an outbreak of acne. Unfortunately due to the spreadability of bacteria, it is not uncommon for a person to experience a larger acne breakout if they mess around with a pustule. The reason for this is because Acne involves the presence of bacteria, which are feeding off the natural oils in the pore of the skin. If the bacteria has plenty of oils to feed off of, and the bacteria gets spread by popping a zit, etc. then the bacteria will find its way into another pore and live there. The bacteria will live in many pores and feed off the oils. The body's natural immune response will kick in and try to destroy the bad bacteria, but in some cases the bacteria is too strong or your natural immune response is weak and then the only way to get rid of, or get under control, the bacteria is to go on antibiotics as prescribed by a Dermatologist.

Antibiotic Truth

It is true antibiotics are wonderful at treating the infestation of bacteria in the skin, but be careful of the use of antibiotics for this topical bacteria treatment. Unless you have severe acne (this is NOT an occasional, or even weekly 5-6 non-cystic zits) you should think carefully about the over prescription of antibiotics and it's potential weakening of your natural immune response to the internal bacteria you may run into down the road. It's the bacteria that lives inside you not on you, that you REALLY need to worry about.

The skin is a marvel of creation. It is a solid protective blanket made up of multiple layers, with only a few orifices to allow penetration inside the body. Because of this, the bacteria that cause pustules and acne are all living in the outer layers of the skin. So there is no worry about the bacteria penetrating deeper into the system, unless YOU force it there by breaking the skin by being too aggressive.

Bacteria, the real deal

Bacteria are a microorganism that feeds off of a host. Bacteria LOVE the oil that lubricates our skin. It also really loves closed, warm, moist areas. So, a closed pore is the perfect breeding ground for bacteria to make lots of babies.

But as gross as this is, know that your skin is covered with surface bacteria. It's there all the time and it doesn't hurt you. It's kind of like spiders, if you drive away one type of spider, you may end up with a worse kind of spider. Same is potentially true for the bacteria on your skin. So, just know it's there. And for the most part it's not a problem, if you keep everything in check.

Pus.............friend or foe?

Pus is gross. It looks weird. It feels weird and it really makes you think of disease. And who wants to walk around looking like a disease freak?

The truth is that pus is not bad at all. It's gotten a really bad rap, but it's really, honestly a good thing. It is doing a very good service for your body and is an important stage in healing the damage your skin is undergoing when under the attack of too much trapped bacteria.

Pus, technically, is a mixture of white blood cells and bacteria. There's probably some other stuff in there too, but basically it's just the bad guys (bacteria) being eaten by the good guys (white blood cells). When you think about it that way, it doesn't seem so bad.

The way it happens is like this: if you get some bacteria in overproduction in your pore, and there is a lot of oil in there too (this is oil coming from the inside out for the most part, so yes, diet does matter) then the bacteria start to overwhelm the pore and begin attacking and irritating the pore lining. This sends a message to your immune system. "Call in the guards!" it screams. And it sends in all these white blood cells to eat away at the overproduction of bacteria.

The other good thing about pus is it keeps the whole pore nice and moist while it's fighting the bacteria, so there isn't as much damage to the pore lining. Skin really likes moisture.

Oil.......ally or enemy?

Why is it that 20 minutes after you wash your face, suddenly that taught skin you had is gone and you feel comparably like a fish fry? It's oil. The body's cool way of keeping itself moisturized and pliable. It's really an important component to healthy, long living skin. But it is about balance. Too much oil and you can have an overproduction of bacteria and then you're experiencing the trickle down effect right into zit-o-pia.

Too little oil and you've got flaky, dry skin that itches and wrinkles and is not healthy on a systemic level, not just on a zit by zit level.

For thousands of years the Ayurvedic tradition in India has utilized oils to manage the vitality and health of the skin. This system uses oils to lubricate and expunge clogged oil deposits, like attracts like and as an Aesthetician I have seen how successful topical application of oils can be in the removal of a clogged dry blackhead plug. I mention this, not to encourage you as the acne or zit sufferer to apply vegetable oil to your skin in the treatment of it, but instead to help raise awareness about how there are specific good oils (jojoba, sesame oil, rose oil) that can help maintain healthy skin.

In the Western culture there is an over proliferation of products which are designed to dry the skin, and although there are times when this is a good idea, there are other times when drying the skin is actually aiding and abetting the destabilization of the health of the skin. So don't give in to the "fight the oil" battle, remember it's about balance. Too much of anything is not a good thing, be it oil or bacteria.

The Solution

How do I get rid of it?

So, now you know what you've got on your hands. How do I get rid of it? Well, if you can wait and be patient. The zit should probably be clear within 8-10 days and be in the plug stage that is A LOT easier to remove. If you can't wait, skim down to the "How to Pop a Zit" step-by-step guide.

Whatever steps you take, you will be well advised to remember the golden rules of prevention:

1. Wash your face daily (but don't over strip! Oil is not your enemy)
2. Massage your face (gently) daily with clean fingers
3. You are what you eat, because hormones contribute to everything.
4. Don't spread the infection! Sterilize your hands and clean the surrounding areas after working with each pustule.

Dangers of Popping

However you look at it, a zit is ugly, but it's nothing compared to the alternatives. A scar is a lifelong reminder of what went terribly wrong because of one little infection. That said, sometimes that zit just has to go, but before you dive in know what you are doing. Read the Step-by-Step guide to avoid the dangers of popping. But here they are, just so you know.

If you pop a pustule without properly opening the "seal" of skin, you're forcing the pus to break the seal, and it will break it in a ripping fashion. Skin doesn't heal serrated rips very well, so it can take longer to heal and cause a weakened healing response, a scar, in the process.

Also, if you use the wrong techniques, you could end up forcing the pus down into the pore, getting it trapped in deeper levels of the dermis, and therefore causing a cyst. A cyst is very difficult to extract manually and should be dealt with by a medical professional who will either prescribe an antibiotic or surgically remove the cyst sac, which could lead to a more aggressive scar.

Step by Step

How to Pop a Zit

BLACKHEAD/non-pus COMEDONE:

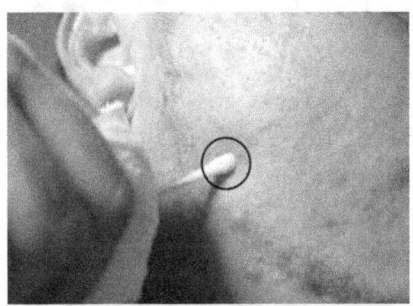

1. Wipe blackhead area with cotton swab soaked in witch hazel.

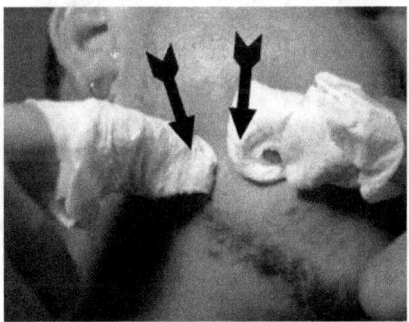

2. Take two pieces of cotton tissue and cover index fingers on both hands. Keep the tissue padded over fingertips. Using your index fingers or a combination of padded index finger and thumb, gently press on skin.

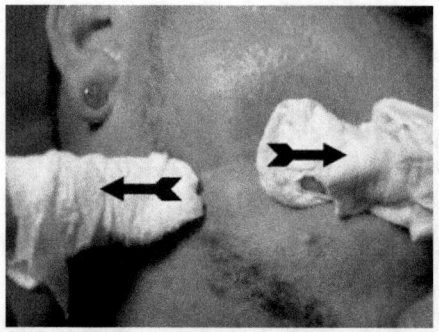

3. Gently press down on the skin surrounding the pore. Approximately 1mm from the pore itself.

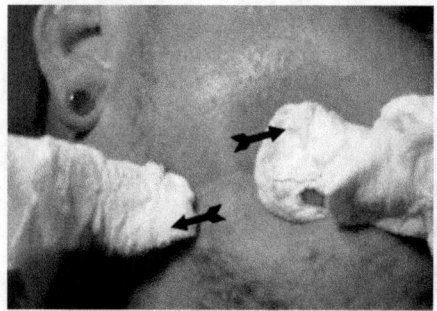

4. While keeping some pressure on the skin, pull skin taught by pulling fingers away from each other. Keep the impacted pore in the center.

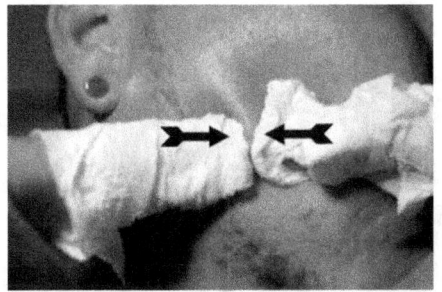

5. While pressing downward, press fingers together, do not let fingers touch each other. Scoop fingers in an upward motion under the impacted pore, while maintaining pressure. Do NOT pinch the skin.

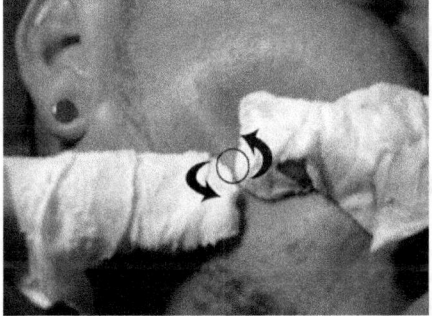

6. Massage around the opening of the pore. Feel free to gently wiggle fingers back and forth while pressing on either side of the blackhead. Don't forget to keep scooping up under the pore.

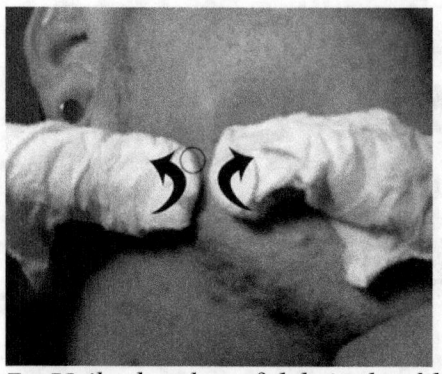

7. Voila the plug of debris should extract itself.

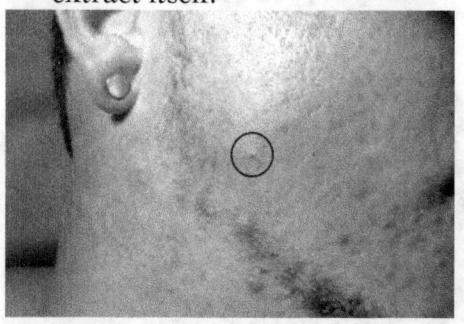

+If this does not work, try more massage around the perimeter of the pore, make sure you do this with clean, sterilized hands or cotton swabs.

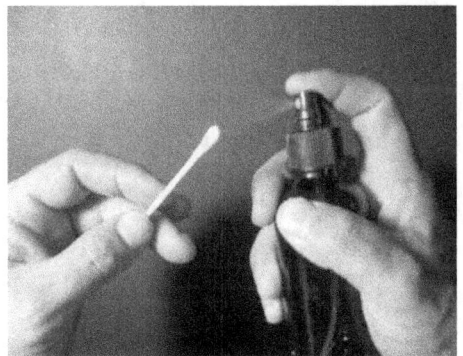

10. Spray Cotton Swab with Hydrogen Peroxide or Witch Hazel.

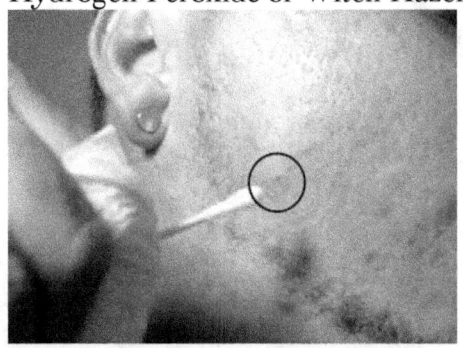

11. Firmly dab wet cotton swab on the extracted pore.

PUSTULE POPPING:

First thing to remember: SANITATION! If you've got a pustule or anything with pus in it, make sure you've got Witch Hazel or Hydrogen Peroxide at the ready. Alcohol is too drying to be applied to the skin, but Witch Hazel will help in the clean up of any straying pus.

1. Moisten cotton swab with witch hazel
2. Wipe moistened cotton swab over pustule
3. Take the thinnest needle you can find (a lancet is ideal) and sterilize the end by running through a burning flame. Allow to cool. Once this step is done do not touch the tip of the needle (for a sterilized lancet skip this step)
4. Clean tip of needle with rubbing alcohol.
5. Insert tip of sterilized needle/lancet SIDEWAYS into the pustule. Do not insert the tip directly down, but instead in a sideways motion, then remove the needle tip without ripping the skin.
6. Take two pieces of cotton tissue and cover index fingers on both hands. Keep the tissue padded over fingertips.
7. Place covered fingertips on skin.

8. Gently pull the skin taught by pulling fingers away from each other.
9. With covered fingers pulled away from the white head press in downward motion.
10. While pressing downward, press fingers together, without actually touching each other.
11. Press fingers in upward motion.
12. Voila! Puss should extract itself through the opening made by the lancet.
13. Be as thorough as possible, without going overboard. Clean out the runny liquid, but be careful to stop at any sign of clear liquid. Any harder plugish material can be extracted and you'll have good results.
14. Wipe off the pus with witch hazel (or Hydrogen Peroxide) soaked cotton swab. Try not to drag pus across face.
15. Ideally take aloe vera gel and dab on top of extracted pustule.

Post-Pop Care

Pustules

You will have a red spot on your face from this, but the bump should be gone so you can cover it with make-up (if ABSOLUTELY NECESSARY). Know that an open wound like the popped pustule should not be covered by make-up but, instead (if absolutely necessary) a silicone cover applied BEFORE the make-up. If you don't do this, you risk feeding the bacteria in the popped pore, by filling it with oily make-up. The best remedy is to pop at night before bed, apply aloe vera gel and let the pore and skin breathe. Oxygen is bacteria's enemy. Consider this a now open wound, and although not bleeding, must be treated with care to avoid long-term damage to the skin and scarring.

1. Don't cover it up: No band-aids or make-up. Let open air help heal the wound. Oxygen is bacteria's worst enemy.

2. Use a topical toner on the pore, like witch hazel, or Hydrogen Peroxide, until the punctured area is no longer "open".

3. Avoid harsh soaps (always do this) or Scrubs. The manual scraping of the skin can cause the punctured area to become ripped even further.

Comedones/ non-pus Blackheads

Because the debris has been allowed to solidify and is no longer spreadable, once you've extracted the plug from the pore and disposed of it, the treatment of the skin is pretty easy. There isn't very much healing that needs to happen. Therefore, simply wipe the plugged area with a witch hazel soaked cotton swab. Let dry. And maintain the basic cleansing procedure for daily skin care. Witch Hazel is an excellent daily toner. It also works as a temporary skin tightener, leaving the pore temporarily reduced. Daily use of Hydrogen Peroxide on the skin can lead to dehydrated pores that leads to sagging skin.

Mahatmama.com who?

www.Mahatmama.com is committed to providing information that helps us, as humans, lead healthier, richer lives. Our conception is based on the Red Tent model: to gather, to support, to nourish and to share. At Mahatmama.com all are welcome to gather in community to bring to light the issues that need addressing, in the hope of finding answers. We support each other to allow free expression within the context of moving forward, to collectively find answers. We nourish one another and our individual role as community members. As guides, we are the ultimate students, and so we share to reach new heights of understanding, comprehension and evolution in our thinking, our living and in our actions with all. Come join the tent.